Why Are You Taking My Tonsils?

PAULA L WHITLEY-MINER RN

ILLUSTRATED BY ALICE C FACENTE RN

ISBN: 1466475889
ISBN-13: 9781466475885

Why Are You Taking My Tonsils?

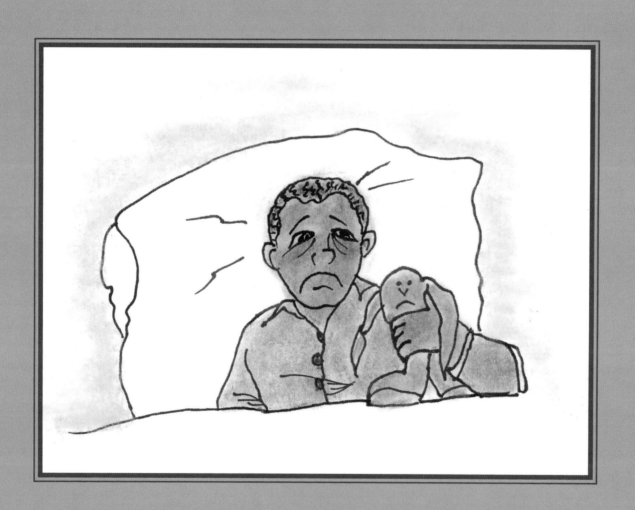

"Not again," Jimmy thought as he rolled onto his belly. Sleep quickly fell away with each sandpaper-like swallow. Drool soaked his pillow; it hurt too much to swallow. His head began to beat like a drum and his cheeks felt hot against the sheets. Goose-bumps ran up and down his body as he pulled his legs up and shivered. He didn't even want to stay home from school again!

"Mom! Dad!" His voice was thick and bloated.

His parents hurried in, already concerned since Jimmy was usually bouncing out of bed, the first to turn on the TV in the morning.

"Jimmy, what's the matter, Honey?" asked his mom as she reached for his forehead, but his pink cheeks already gave away the fever she felt.

"This has been happening for months now. Jimmy needs to have his throat checked by a doctor. He's been sick too much and shouldn't miss any more school," decided Jimmy's dad.

Later, Jimmy, snuggling deep into the pillows on the couch, was watching colorful cartoons dance across the TV. His fever was down after taking the medicine his mom gave him. He didn't like taking medicine because it hurt to swallow, but he took it and now he felt better.

"Keep drinking the cold water," his mother called to him from the kitchen. "It will help your throat."

Jimmy still wasn't talking much. His voice sounded like he imagined a frog would sound, the kind with the big balloon neck.

"We are going to a new doctor today to have your throat checked," his mother told him.

"Why a new doctor? I like my doctor," croaked Jimmy from the backseat of the car as they drove to the new doctor's office.

"Well, I like your doctor too, but he wants you to be checked by a new doctor who takes care of kids who get a lot of sore throats, like you," explained Jimmy's mom as they walked into the doctor's office.

"Jimmy, you have tonsillitis," explained Dr. Stephens as he sat with Jimmy and his mom.

"What's that?" he questioned.

"Tonsillitis is the swelling and infection of the tonsils," continued Dr. Stephens. "The tonsils are in the back of your throat, Jimmy. They help to clean your body of germs, but sometimes they become unable to work properly and need to be removed. Your mom said you have often been sick with a fever, aches, trouble swallowing, trouble breathing through your nose, and a very sore throat."

"I also had trouble hearing and my voice sounded different. Mom and Dad say I've even snored at night!" exclaimed Jimmy.

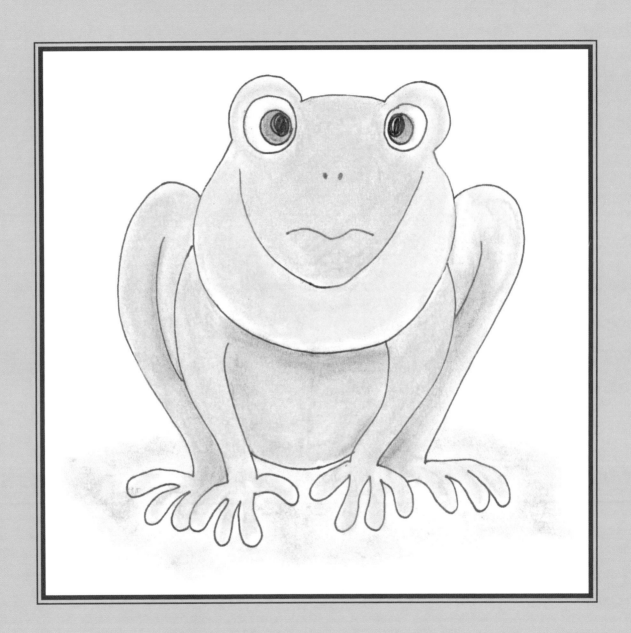

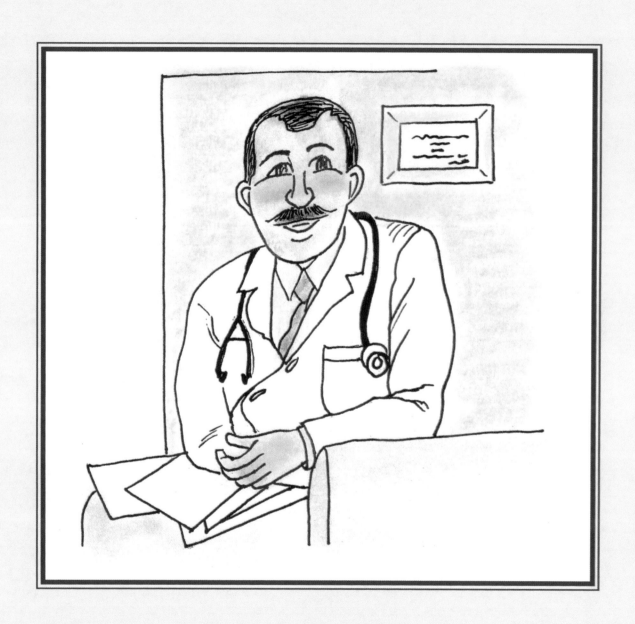

"Sometimes your hearing is affected when the adenoids become swollen. The adenoids, like the tonsils, try to clean your body of germs and are above and behind the uvula in the back of your throat," Dr. Stephens explained further.

Jimmy looked at his mom and Dr. Stephens, "My third grade teacher even moved my seat to the front of the class because I couldn't hear her."

"Well, you have been sick a lot this school year. The tonsillitis has affected your learning at school," said Jimmy's mom.

"What do you think, Doctor Stephens?" she asked.

"It's time for them to come out," Doctor Stephens decided.

Jimmy's eyes widened as his mom and Doctor Stephens talked. Tonsillectomy and Adenoidectomy! An operation in the hospital! Jimmy's stomach did flip flops! What did it all mean?

The next week, after school, Jimmy's mom and dad brought him to the hospital. They told him today's visit was for them to see where to go and what to expect when Jimmy had his tonsils and adenoids removed. Jimmy's stomach started to feel jumpy again. He saw a lady in a uniform walking over to them. Jimmy squeezed his parents' hands.

"Welcome to Same Day Surgery. You must be Jimmy. My name is Ann. I am a nurse here and I'd like to show you and your parents around." Jimmy looked up at the nurse's smiling face. She seemed nice, so Jimmy smiled too.

"I have a question," Jimmy stated.

"Well, what's your first question, Jimmy?"

Nurse Ann kneeled down to talk to Jimmy.

He liked not having to look up.

"What does Same Day Surgery mean?" asked Jimmy.

"It means that you come here in the morning, have your operation and then go home later the same day," explained Nurse Ann.

Nurse Ann walked with Jimmy and his parents through a door that opened by itself and into a long hallway. Pretty cool, thought Jimmy, but he still had some butterflies in his tummy as he walked through the door holding his mom and dad's hands. He saw a lot of pretty little bedrooms. As he looked closer, each room had its own TV and the few people in the beds were either asleep, visiting with family or watching TV. A few even waved to him. He shyly waved back. Other people dressed like Nurse Ann, walked back and forth between the rooms.

"Who are all these people?" Jimmy asked wide-eyed.

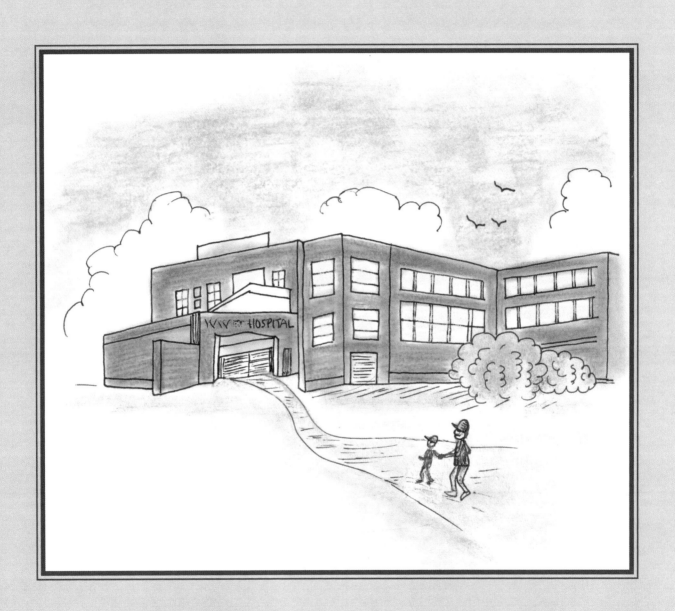

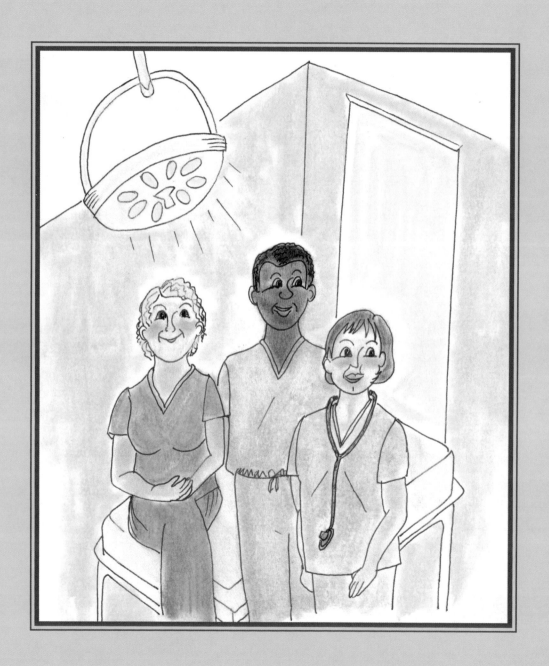

"These are people who are trained in taking care of someone having an operation. Some are the doctors who actually do the surgery. We also have doctors who help you fall asleep and stay asleep during the surgery," explained Nurse Ann. "We also have nurses and technicians who take care of you and assist the doctors. Some nurses will take care of you before the surgery and some nurses will take care of you after the surgery and get you ready to go home," she continued.

"I want my mom and dad to stay with me when I come here," said Jimmy.

"Your parents will be with you while you are waiting for your operation and one parent can even go into the operating room while you fall asleep. They will be with you in the recovery room as you wake up. The recovery room is the room you wake up in after the operation. Then once you are awake, you and your parents will come back here to Same Day Surgery to start getting ready to go home. Your parents will have to wear a funny outfit while in the operating room though," explained Nurse Ann.

"Why do they have to wear special clothes?" asked Jimmy.

"Everyone wears special clothes to keep germs out of the Operating Room and all the equipment used is specially cleaned - we call it sterilization - to make sure you are healthy after your surgery," explained Nurse Ann.

Jimmy, still holding his parents' hands, felt his stomach butterflies lighten and continued walking with Nurse Ann.

"You'll probably have to wake up early the morning of your surgery Jimmy, but you cannot eat or drink anything. It's very important that you not eat or drink because of the anesthesia. Anesthesia is the medicine that makes you fall asleep while Dr. Stephens takes out your tonsils and adenoids, and it can make your stomach upset," informed Nurse Ann as they stopped by one of the little bedrooms.

"This is one of our rooms where we will have you change into our pajamas and get you ready to go to the operating room," explained Nurse Ann as she and Jimmy sat on the comfy bed.

"What do you have to do?" asked Jimmy as he looked around at the TV-like screens.

"Well, the doctors and the nurses will ask your mom and dad about your health. One of the nurses will give you some medicine to drink that might make you sleepy and will help you be comfortable after surgery. Soon after, a nurse from the operating room will bring you and one of your parents to your operating room. Jimmy, you will get a special hat to wear to keep germs away, and your mom or dad will be wearing the special outfit. When you get into the operating room, you breathe into a mask, it might smell like grapes, and the medicine you breathe in will make you fall asleep. Then Dr. Stephens will take out your tonsils and adenoids. You won't even know it," smiled Nurse Ann.

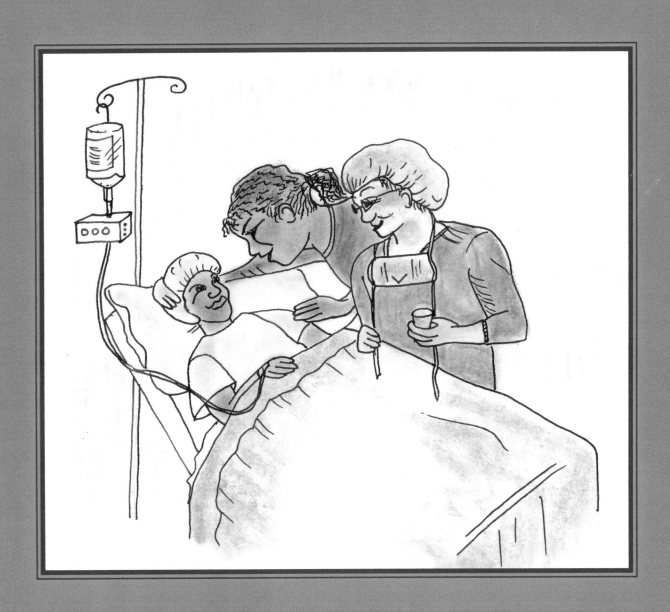

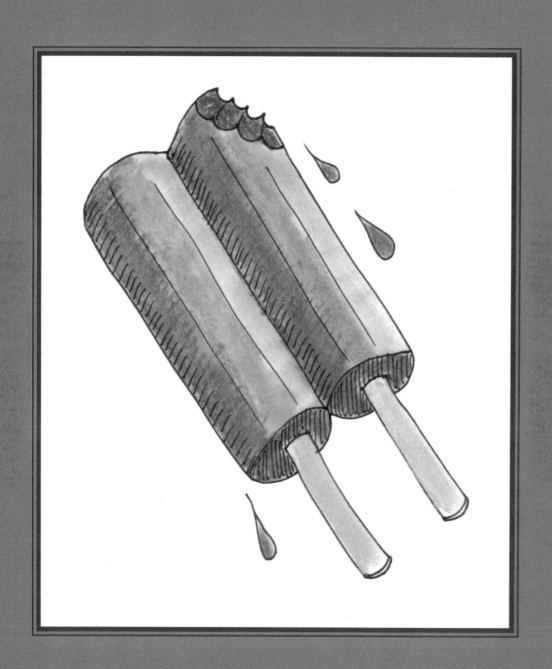

"And then I`ll wake up in the recovery room?" remembered Jimmy.

"That's right, you'll wake up in the recovery room and your mom or dad will be with you. You might see a plastic bag hanging upside down with a tube in your hand. That is an IV, an intravenous line, it will be in your hand giving fluids to your body while you are asleep. We know your throat may be sore. We'll give you medicine to make it feel better as well as some cool liquids to drink when you are awake enough. Once you are drinking and steady on your feet, you might feel a little wobbly at first, we'll be able to send you home," Nurse Ann continued.

"Will my throat hurt a lot?" Jimmy asked.

"Well, Jimmy, your throat is going to hurt and that's the truth, but there are ways to make your throat hurt less. Doctor Stephens and your nurse will talk with you and your parents about how to take care of yourself when you go home from the hospital. It's good that you came here today so you know what to expect and so you can prepare for after the surgery," smiled Nurse Ann.

"How do I do that?" wondered Jimmy.

"You can go to the store before the surgery and pick out special cool drinks and frozen treats you might like to have when you go home. When you are home after the surgery, it is important for you to drink or eat these frozen treats to keep your throat wet - that will make your throat hurt less. Frequent small sips are best. Maybe pick out some movies to watch while you are resting at home. Before your surgery, your parents can pick up the special sore throat medicine you will need. That way when you leave the hospital you can go right home. Take your pain medicine regularly because that will make you feel better and then you can drink more. I know you probably don't take naps anymore but that is also a good thing to do because naps help your body," explained Nurse Ann.

"We talked about a lot during your visit today Jimmy and I have a question for you now. Do you remember the things you should do to make yourself feel better after your surgery?" Nurse Ann asked Jimmy.

"Take my medicine, drink and rest," answered Jimmy immediately.

"Excellent, Jimmy! You will do great when you have your surgery," laughed Nurse Ann.

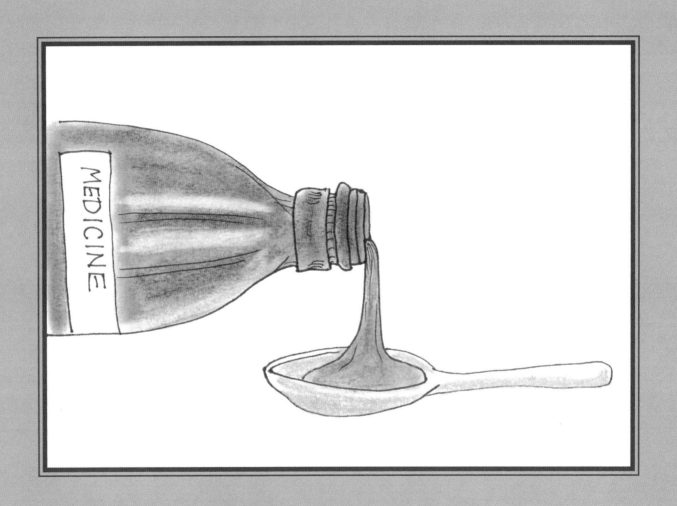

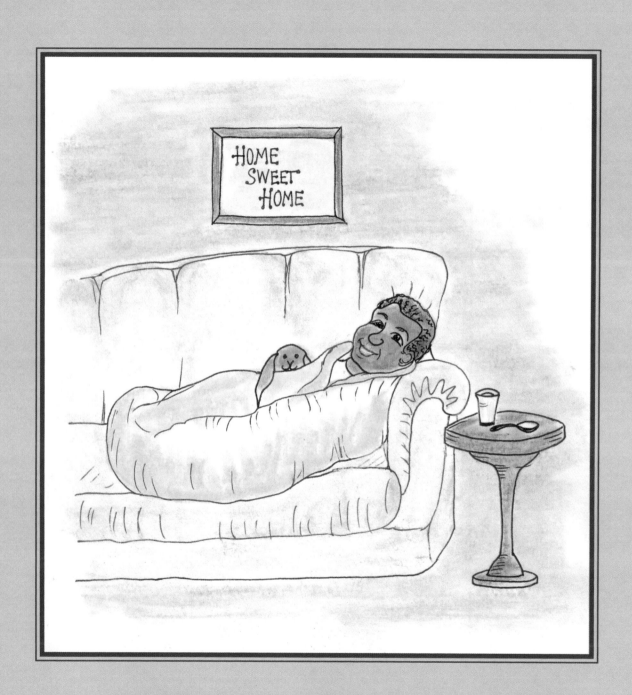

Jimmy's stomach didn't do anymore flip flops. He and his parents were comfortable and prepared for his surgery later that week. He saw his friends Nurse Ann and Dr. Stephens. He remembered what he learned when he had visited the hospital and he and his parents had everything ready at home. He even put one of his favorite blankets on the couch to wait for him.

He stayed home for about a week after the operation, but when he went back to school he brought his hospital hat and bracelet to show his third grade friends and told them all about his big adventure.

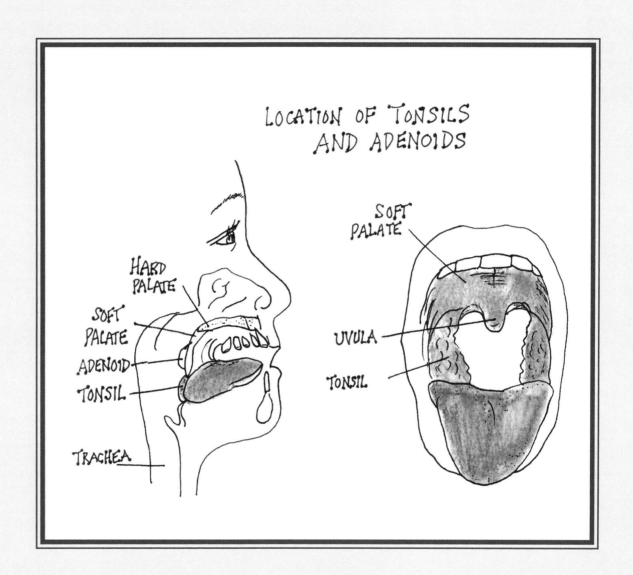

LOCATION OF TONSILS AND ADENOIDS

HARD PALATE

SOFT PALATE

SOFT PALATE

ADENOID

UVULA

TONSIL

TONSIL

TRACHEA

PRE-PROCEDURE

- Talk with child in calm, reassuring manner.
- Check with surgical center if tours are offered and take tour.
- Register and complete any required blood-work at surgical center days ahead of time.
- No aspirin or Motrin (ibuprofen) products for 10 days before the surgery. Tylenol is acceptable.
- Ask for and fill prescriptions before the surgery.
- If the child becomes sick the day before or the day of surgery call the surgeon.
- Child may bring in favorite stuffed animal, toy or blanket to hold in surgical center.
- Leave valuables at home.
- Wear comfortable clothes - parents too.
- Child cannot eat or drink: Parents, do not eat or drink in front of child, but do eat something.

POST-PROCEDURE

- Go straight home after the surgery.
- Frequent cool or room-temperature fluids. At least ½ cup of fluid every hour while awake. For example - ice water, Italian ice, sherbet, ice cream (if makes phlegmy and needs to keep clearing throat then don't take), apple sauce, yogurt, pudding. Keep cool water at bedside during night.
- As time passes, a day or so, try advancing diet, for example - scrambled eggs cooled and chopped, mini-pasta dish cooled (no tomato products).
- Usually a regular diet can be resumed in about 1 week.
- Watch for dehydration - if little or no fluids are taken in 24 hours call the surgeon. Signs of dehydration include lethargy and reduced or very concentrated urine output.
- Fever greater than 101.5 degrees - may indicate dehydration or infection: call the surgeon.
- Rest with head elevated to decrease swelling.
- An ice collar to front of throat can be helpful.

- Pain medications can be nauseating, take with food, i.e. pudding.
- If persistent nausea and vomiting develop, call surgeon.
- Pain medications are more effective when taken before severe pain develops, take them regularly but not more frequently than prescribed. The more comfortable the child is, the more the child should be able to drink and then feel better.
- Pain can be more problematic at night when there are no other distractions. Try to time pain medication for bedtime.
- Child may complain of referred ear pain.
- Watch for bleeding. Bleeding is rare but can occur usually right after the surgery or 5-10 days later when the scabs that had formed over the tonsil beds fall off and the tissue is raw again. The adenoids are up in back of

oropharynx and if they bleed tend to cause a bloody nose. The tonsil beds can bleed and drip down the throat and cause vomiting. Blood does not settle in the stomach and usually comes back up.

- Look at the vomit to see if it is bright red fresh blood or old dark brown that could have settled in the stomach during the surgery. Call the surgeon if there is any question of bleeding. Ice water mouth washes may help. If there is severe bleeding, go to the nearest Emergency Department.
- Remember to call the surgeon if there are any questions or concerns. Reach the surgeon by calling the office phone number 24 hours a day.

SCRAP BOOK PAGE

Picture in hospital bed

Picture in hospital bed

Pre-op

Post-op

Picture resting at home

Hospital bracelet

REFERENCES

Burden, Nancy. *Ambulatory Surgical Nursing (second edition).* Philadelphia, PA, W.B. Saunders Company, 2000.

Healthwise Inc. "Tonsillitis Surgery." (Online) Available http://www.webmd.com/oral-health/tc/tonsillitis-surgery June 11, 2011.

Kalantar, Nader and Takehana, Christopher. "Shorter Post-operative Recovery Stay Following Outpatient Tonsillectomy is Safe, Cost-efficient." (Online) Available: http://www.medicalnewstoday.com/releases/56962.php November, 2006.

MedicineNet.com. "Tonsillectomy and Adenoidectomy Surgical Instruction." (Online) Available: http://www.medicinenet.com/tonsillectomy/article.htm 27 September, 2002.

Miller MD, Benjamin F. and Kean, Claire, RN, B.S., M.Ed. *Encyclopedia and Dictionary of Medicine, Nursing, and Allied Health.* Philadelphia, PA: W B Saunders Co, 1978.

31576324R00019

Made in the USA
Lexington, KY
16 April 2014